SEX POSITIONS MASTERY

100 TOP SEX POSITIONS TO MAKE HER SCREAM!

A second editiono title by **Madleine Carter**

CONTENTS

ABOUT THE AUTHOR

Madeleine Carter is a self-made entrepreneur, author, publisher and successful academic. Having founded the SexMastery.com and completing her academic career, Anastasia turned her attention to using her experience and skills to become a respected author and reviewer among the community.

Anastasia has been publishing on Kindle and on various other platforms for several years now. Her work can be found on Kindle, Createspace and Lulu as either ebooks or as paperbacks. Her books are available as paperbacks and as e-books for you to read on Kindle Cloud Reader on your computer, or on your tablet/other mobile device.

Check out her author page to view the whole range of content that she has available to you and keep up to date with the most recent promotions, deals and free offers that are often available to you.

amazon.com/author/madeleinecarter

PART I - ORGASMS

HOW TO MAKE HER COME

We all know by now that you have to work to get a girl to orgasm, and I mean a genuine orgasm. The sad truth is that most women end up faking an orgasm to avoid the awkward tension she knows that he hasn't got her there. But no one should have to resort to this; it should never be an option. Period.

The orgasm isn't purely physical; the emotional and psychological elements are still so, so important. It's possible for a person to orgasm without even being touched. It's hard, sure, but it is certainly possible. I just need to demonstrate to you the significance of the mind here. It's a key part to getting a female to her ultimate climax. Think about tantric sex. Now, you might not know a lot about tantric sex, but the idea is that sex is considered spiritual in nature – it's linked to a higher state of being. So clearly sex is more than the mere physical act of stimulating the nerves.

It's important to remember that sex, like I will keep reminding you throughout this discussion, is about a lot more than the physical act. I'm sure you've heard the saying that sex is 10% physical and 90% in the mind. I know this might be a little hard to believe at first. The best sex should be an expression of how you feel towards your partner. This doesn't mean that it needs to be super slow and passionate throughout – you can still show your girl how you feel by having fun.

Moving on, I mentioned earlier about how there are multiple ways to bring a girl to orgasm. There's the vaginal orgasm, there's the clitoral orgasm, or you can even bring a girl to orgasm through anal sex or without even touching her! But we'll get on to this later. Firstly, I want to talk about vaginal orgasms and clitoral orgasms. The quite sad reality is that a lot of women very rarely experience vaginal orgasms, but rather find that clitoral stimulation is the only way they ever have been able to reach climax. That's why a lot of guys tend to focus greatly on stimulating a clitoral orgasm because it's generally a lot easier and a lot more reliable. None-the-less, it's important not to disregard other orgasms that a female can come to and understand how and why a female comes to such an orgasm.

Not all women reach orgasm in the same way and not all women will reach orgasm every time they have sex. Some women need direct clitoral stimulation to reach an orgasm, while others can have clitoral orgasms through direct clitoral stimulation and/ or sexual intercourse. This means that before you start even trying to reach orgasm, you have to experiment. You need to understand what you need from your partner and what your partner needs from you to reach an orgasm. After a few experiments, you should have a pretty good idea of how to get there.

If you find that clitoral stimulation is needed to reach orgasm, make sure you and your partner focus largely on foreplay. This will turn you both on and get you ready for sex and is a great way to bond with your partner to increase your chances of reaching an orgasm. Use whatever feels best – physical, oral or even a vibrator can massively increase your chances of getting there before sex. During intercourse, you should try positions that allow easy access to the clitoris, like cowgirl or spooning.

If you need clitoral stimulation through intercourse, try altered missionary positions. Try starting off in the missionary position, bring your legs together between your partners and have him shit his weight so that pressure is applied to the clitoris when he thrusts.

If you need G-spot stimulation, the G spot is located on the front wall of the vagina. You will need to find the right angles and positions that allow deep penetration. Try missionary or doggy style. Reverse cowgirl is also a great position which allows you to control penetration depth and the angle you need to stimulate the G-spot.

We all know that women can orgasm, obviously. But a lot of guys are confused when it comes to a female coming. Girl's often will tell you 'I just came', and they probably did. But what confuses a lot of guys is that women can ejaculate just like them! It's normal and it's great. For whatever reason, this seems to baffle a lot of people because it just doesn't make sense to them and think that it might just be some sort of myth that has been made in the spotlight of pornography, but it's very, very real.

And what's great is that if you've brought a female to ejaculation you know that you've done well. Female ejaculation is the highlight of the female orgasm and is one of the most pleasurable sensations a person can feel. It's on par with full body convulsions and eye-rolling orgasms.

The most common signals that will tell you is a girl is coming can be seen by the way she acts. She will likely start moving with less control, her eyes might drift upwards and she will moan uncontrollably. But a lot of this is easily faked – I'm sure you've read a lot about fake orgasms and how so many women pretend to come. It shouldn't be this way, but it is. Now it's up to you to make sure that your partner never feels the need to fake again because you're genuinely making her scream!

Which brings us to squirting. It's one thing that simply can't be faked and guarantees that she really is having an amazing time. If she doesn't, don't be too disheartened because it can take time to get to know exactly what each individual girl likes, and some find it easier than others to get to the point where they can squirt. Just note that they are generally caused by a combination of clitoral stimulation and G-spot stimulation. Mix it up, find out and be responsive like always.

It can take around 20 minutes to get a female to orgasm and you should start with foreplay. Although general guidelines, there is a reason why these are such good ones. If you want to reach a squirting orgasm, the time needs to be put in to really heat things up before you even have intercourse. If successful here, then the chances are that she won't have anything to say – she will quite literally be speechless! When females experience such a hard orgasm, they physically won't be able to say anything! They will be so overwhelmed by the sensation that there is no need for words.

Finally, we should talk about the most talked about the difference between guys and girls. Guys come, great! Buuuuut, there are limitations. Once a guy has come, he is physically unable to come again – there is a short period, around 20-30 minutes, where it is genuinely impossible for a guy to get hard again. It's a whole other story for women. Women are able to have multiple orgasms over and over again. Women are massively blessed when it comes to sex. When it 'comes' to giving a girl multiple orgasms, it's generally easier to make her come the second time than it is to make her come the first time! If orgasm is reached one way, change things up to try and get to a second orgasm another way. If it doesn't work, go back to the first way and try again.

HOW TO HAVE A
BETTER ORGASM

This section has a fair bit to do with the last chapter, so I'm not going to go in too deep here (pun intended). You've probably met, or at least heard about, women that always find it so hard to have a complete orgasm or even those who have never, ever orgasmed! This comes across as such sad news because it shouldn't have to be this way. We are a highly sexual species and amongst the only species that have sex for pleasure – we literally go out of our way to experience the best physical and emotional sensation we can, so why do we often fall short of this goal?

Again, I need to point out that guys and girls are different. Both can have immense pleasure from sex, but girls undoubtedly get the better deal because they have the ability to have multiple orgasms. As a male, you simply can't.

So, how can a girl reach multiple orgasms? I went over this briefly in the last chapter, but you are going to want to switch between clitoral stimulation and the G-spot each time she comes. You're going to need to repeat this over and over again and you could give her orgasm after orgasm! If you put in the time to do this, she will be mind-blown by you and reward you back in return. The better the time she's having, the better the time you're going to have.

PART II - 101 SEX POSITIONS

MAN TRAP

This is a variation of the missionary position. The female should lie back on a bed in the missionary position and have the male lay on top. As he begins to thrust, the female can wrap her legs around him and have more control over the speed and pace of sex.

This is great if you just want some simple sex. You can put little twists on the move like arching the back for better stimulation. Wrapping the legs around the male will also get him going a lot faster!

1. The female should lie on her back in the missionary position – legs open wide and slightly bent.

2. The male should position himself over the female and face her.

3. The male can then penetrate the vagina, just as in the ordinary missionary position.

4. As the male begins thrusting, or when it feels best, the female can wrap her legs around the male and 'trap' him, forcing him closer of allowing some extra room for him to re-position.

5. Tip: Using a pillow under the female's back can help

cause an arch. This will greatly increase pleasure and will make things much more comfortable when wrapping her legs around the male.

Safety Tips

This position can cause a lot of strain on the female's lower back, so make sure support is provided by using a pillow or cushion! Be sure to ask whether your partner is comfortable and not in any pain at any point and don't be ashamed if you need to say something because *you* are uncomfortable!

THE DECKCHAIR

The male should sit on the bed with his legs stretched out and his hands behind him to support his own weight. He should lean back and bend his elbows slightly. The female should then lie back on a pillow facing him and put her feet up on to his shoulders. She can then move her hips forwards and back and begin having sex.

This is an amazing position for very deep penetration for G-spot stimulation.

1. The male should sit on a bed with his legs stretched out. He can use his hands behind him to support his weight.

2. He should then carefully lean back and bend his elbows slightly for further support and control.

3. The female should then position herself by the male's feet, facing him and laying back on a pillow for support.

4. Once in position, the female can begin moving herself closer towards the male until her feet are up on his shoulders.

5. Finally, she can move her hips towards his penis for insertion.

6. In this position, once penetrated, it is best for the female to be in control and thrust her hips back and forth to get the best control and stimulation.

Safety Tips

This position can cause a lot of strain on the female's lower back, so make sure support is provided by using a pillow or cushion! Be sure to ask whether your partner is comfortable and not in any pain at any point and don't be ashamed if you need to say something because *you* are uncomfortable!

CORRIDOR COSY

This one can be tricky as you need to be in an enclosed area. The male needs to lean against a wall and needs to shuffle his way towards the floor until his feet are touching an opposing wall. The female should climb down on top of his legs, supporting her own weight. Her legs should be left dangling and she can begin thrusting.

This is a great one for adventurous and exciting sex!

1. Find an enclosed area with secure structures such as a thin corridor, hallway, or other appropriate settings.

2. The male should lean against one side of the wall and lower himself carefully by extending his legs outwards to the opposing wall.

3. IMPORTANT: The male's feet should always remain on the floor and securely in place at the base of the opposing wall.

4. The female should position herself on top of him and

face towards him.

5. The female can begin lowering herself towards the penis for penetration, using either the walls around her or the male's shoulders for support. The female's legs should be left dangling while she is on top.

6. Finally, she can begin thrusting back and forth.

7. Tip: If this position is too taxing on the strength of either the male or the female, consider having the male position himself in a lower position so that the female's legs can reach the floor. She can then use her legs to help support her own weight.

Safety Tips

The male needs to make sure that he can support his partner's weight and that he isn't going to slip and fall to the floor completely. Likewise, the female should support her own weight as best she can to avoid potential injury.

TWISTER
STALEMATE

The female should begin by laying on her back with her legs apart. Her partner should kneel down on all fours in between her legs. The female should then lift herself up, wrapping her arms around his chest for support. She should then slowly bring up her legs, so her feet are flat on the bed.

This is a great position for deep penetration and stimulating the G-spot!

1. The female should lie down on her back with her legs apart and slightly bent at the knee.

2. The male should then position himself in-between her legs, facing her and on all fours i.e. on his hands and feet.

3. The female should then wrap her arms up around the male's chest for support. This will require some strength from the female.

4. The female can then bend her legs and begin to raise

her hips. Her feet should now be flat on the bed.

5. Finally, she can guide the penis into her vagina for penetration.

Safety Tips

This position requires some upper body strength from the female. She should make sure to be holding on tightly to her partner as he thrusts.

THE SPIDER

You should start by facing each other. The female should climb on to her partner's lap and allow penetration. Her legs should be bent on either side of him and the male should be doing the same. The female should lay back first, slowly followed by the male, until both heads are on the bed. Now, move slowly and calmly.

This is a great one for slow sex to enhance stimulation before trying to reach climax – a good one if you have a lot of time.

1. Both the male and female should begin by sitting on a bed and facing towards each other.

2. The female should then shuffle forward and sit on her partner's lap.

3. This is the point where penetration should occur. The female must remain on top of her partner's lap.

4. Once penetrated, the female should slowly lean backwards and bend her back until her head is on the bed. Her arms can then be positioned outwards until comfortable.

5. The male should repeat this stage, leaning back

slowly until his head is on the bed.

6. The female can then begin thrusting forwards and backwards.

Safety Tips

This position requires penile flexibility, else there is a risk of the male straining his suspensory ligaments!

If you want to find out if the male's penis is flexible enough, have him stand against a wall. Pull his penis gradually down. If the penis is able to point directly down to the ground without causing pain then you should be fine to perform this position, but still be careful.

The female should stay still when the male is initially penetrating her and guide the penis to the vagina. The female should wait while he finds the most comfortable position and angle to thrust without injury.

SPEED BUMP

The female should lay on her stomach and spread her legs. The male should then enter from behind.

The benefit of this position is that things can heat up and speed up very quickly. It is a great position for getting a little rough or if you're having a quickie!

1. The female should lay down on her stomach and spread her legs as wide as she can whilst remaining comfortable.

2. The male should position himself on top of the female with the aim of penetrating from behind, both facing the same way.

3. Once in the position, the male should use his arms to support his weight while he guides his penis towards her vagina for penetration.

4. Finally, the male can perform upwards and downwards thrusts.

Safety Tips

This position can cause a lot of strain on the female's lower back, so make sure support is provided by using a pillow or cushion! Be sure to ask whether your partner is comfortable and not in any pain at any point and don't be ashamed if you need to say something because *you* are uncomfortable!

TRIUMPH ARCH

The male should sit down with his legs stretched out straight. The female should straddle him with her legs either side and kneel down over his penis. Once she has been penetrated, she can lean back until laying down on his legs.

This position can give the female a great orgasm and the male is able to stimulate her clitoris during sex.

1. The male should sit down on a bed with his legs stretched out and straight.

2. The female should straddle over the male, bending her knees until over his penis.

3. Once in position and penetrated, the female can slowly lean back until she is laying down on his legs.

Safety Tips

This position requires penile flexibility, else there is a risk of the male straining his suspensory ligaments!

If you want to find out if the male's penis is flexible

enough, have him stand against a wall. Pull his penis gradually down. If the penis is able to point directly down to the ground without causing pain then you should be fine to perform this position, but still be careful.

The female should stay still when the male is initially penetrating her and guide the penis to the vagina. The female should wait while he finds the most comfortable position and angle to thrust without injury.

THE STANDING WHEELBARROW

For this position, begin in the doggy style position and have the female rest her forearms on some pillows. Her partner should kneel down behind her with one knee bent up to keep himself steady. Once he has penetrated, he should hold her legs and slowly lift her up as he stands.

This position is great if you are just experimenting and just having fun! Otherwise, it is a bit difficult and isn't very well rated for sensation.

1. The female should begin on her hand and knees, facing away from the male (the doggy style position).

2. The female can lean her upper body down towards the floor and rest her forearms on a pillow.

3. The male should kneel down behind her with one knee bent for extra support.

4. He can then position himself towards her for penetration from behind.

5. Finally, the male should grab hold of the female's legs, wherever comfortable and secure, and support her weight as he carefully raises to a standing position.

6. He can then thrust forward and back.

Safety Tips

The male should keep his knees slightly bent when thrusting. If either of you feels uncomfortable during the position, then you should let the other know and try something else! This one isn't for you.

SULTRY SADDLE

In this position, the male lays down on his back with his legs bent and apart – the standard position when the male is on the bottom. The female should slide herself between his legs, almost at a right angle to his body. For support, one hand should be placed on his chest, the other on his leg.

This position relies on the female rocking back and forth until she can feel him hitting her G-spot. The great thing about this position is that the female is completely in control so is one of the better one if G-spot stimulation is what you need to reach an orgasm.

1. The male should lie down on a bed on his back, facing upwards. His legs should be bent at the knee and apart.

2. The female should position herself over the male on her feet or knees, whichever is most comfortable.

3. She can then lower herself to allow for penetration.

4. Once penetrated, the female should place one hand on the male's leg, and the other on his chest for support. She can then use these supports to help her

thrust and control her stimulation.

Safety Tips

This position can cause a lot of strain on the female's lower back, so make sure support is provided by using a pillow or cushion! Be sure to ask whether your partner is comfortable and not in any pain at any point and don't be ashamed if you need to say something because *you* are uncomfortable!

THE PROPELLER

The female should lay on her back with her legs straight and together. The male should lie down on top but be facing down towards her feet. Once penetrated, the male should make small motions with his hips instead of thrusting.

This is a very difficult position and takes some practice to master!

1. The female should lie on her back with her legs straight and together.

2. The male should position himself on top of her in the 180-missionary position i.e. over the female but be facing her feet. He should, as usual, be using his arms for support to hold his body weight.

3. The male can then shuffle backwards until he is able to penetrate the female.

4. Once penetrated, rather than thrusting back and forth, the male should rotate his hips in small circular motions in a 'propeller'-like movement.

Safety Tips

This position requires penile flexibility, else there is a risk of the male straining his suspensory ligaments!

If you want to find out if the male's penis is flexible enough, have him stand against a wall. Pull his penis gradually down. If the penis is able to point directly down to the ground without causing pain then you should be fine to perform this position, but still be careful.

The female should stay still when the male is initially penetrating her and guide the penis to the vagina. The female should wait while he finds the most comfortable position and angle to thrust without injury.

THE LUSTFUL LEG

S tart by standing close and facing each other. The female should have one leg on the bed and the other on top of the male's shoulder, whilst wrapping her arms around his back and neck for support. Then he should carefully penetrate.

Once in position, this is a great move that feels fantastic! It does, however, require some endurance.

1. Both the male and female should begin by standing up beside a bed and facing one another.

2. The female should wrap her arms around the male's neck and shoulders for support.

3. The female can then raise one leg on to the edge of the bed. The other leg can then be raised up to the male's shoulder.

4. Once in position, penetration can take place.

Safety Tips

This position requires penile flexibility to avoid the risk of the male straining his suspensory ligaments!

If you want to find out if the male's penis is flexible enough, have him stand against a wall. Pull his penis gradually down. If the penis is able to point directly down to the ground without causing pain then you should be fine to perform this position, but still be careful.

The female should stay still when the male is initially penetrating her and guide the penis to the vagina. The female should wait while he finds the most comfortable position and angle to thrust without injury.

THE WATERFALL

The male should sit in a sturdy chair. The female can then climb on top with her legs either side of him. She should lean back until her head is on the floor.

The clitoris is very accessible in this position so is great for stimulation during sex. There is also a lot of friction inside the vagina, so this is a great all-rounder for reaching orgasm.

1. The male should find a secure chair and sit on it.

2. The female can then position herself facing towards the male with her legs either side of him.

3. The female should then lower herself on to his penis for penetration.

4. Once inserted, the male should use his hands to support the female behind her back and bottom.

5. The female should then slowly lean backwards until her head is on the floor.

6. Whilst performing step 5 above, the male should take care to support the female's weight however necessary, and the female should take care to move

slowly to ensure that the male is not experiencing any strain or discomfort.

Safety Tips

This position requires penile flexibility, else there is a risk of the male straining his suspensory ligaments!

If you want to find out if the male's penis is flexible enough, have him stand against a wall. Pull his penis gradually down. If the penis is able to point directly down to the ground without causing pain then you should be fine to perform this position, but still be careful.

The female should stay still when the male is initially penetrating her and guide the penis to the vagina. The female should wait while he finds the most comfortable position and angle to thrust without injury.

A pillow should also be used on the floor to support and give comfort to the female's head during sex.

THE CHALLENGE

This is a difficult position (hence the name) and shouldn't be attempted unless you are confident and have tried lots of different positions before – it requires strength and flexibility.

The female should stand on a chair and bend her knees until in the sitting position. She should lean forward with her elbows on her knees. The male should then enter her from behind.

This one is hard to master. If it is too hard for you, you could also have the female simply stand on the ground and lean forward on to a chair as shown in the illustration below.

1. A sturdy and secure chair should be found for this position. It may be useful for the chair to be against a wall.

2. The female should mount the chair and stand up, facing towards the back of the chair and away from the male.

3. She should then carefully bend her knees until in a sitting position.

4. The female should then place her elbows on her knees and hold on to the back of the chair with her hands for support.

5. Finally, once comfortably in position, the male should approach the female from behind for penetration.

Safety Tips

Make sure the chair is very sturdy and you have good footing. The male should support the female throughout and should have a firm hold of the female's waist to keep her steady.

THE SUPERNOVA

For this position, the female should begin on top of the male on a bed or other comfortable place. The male should have his head near the edge. The female should place her feet either side of him and allow penetration by squatting down on his penis. She can then lean back on to her arms behind her.

The female should rock back and forth until she can feel herself reaching climax. When reaching climax, she should lean forward on to her knees and shift the male's upper body off the edge of the bed until she reaches orgasm.

This position is all about timing, but if done right can be really fun and give a great orgasm.

1. The male should begin by lying down, facing upwards and with his knees slightly bent and apart. His head should be near the edge of the bed.

2. The female should place her feet either side of the male's waist and squat down in a straddle position for penetration to take place.

3. The female should then place her hands and arms be-

hind her on the bed and lean backwards. Her arms should be locked and providing most of the support.

4.   She can then begin thrusting back and forth.

5.   When approaching orgasm, the female should launch her upper body forward and on to her knees. This should slightly shuffle the male's head and upper body off of the bed.

6.   Tip: Ensure that the timing is right with the once – it might take some practice. But, once done correctly, this can lead to a fantastic orgasm.

PIRATE'S BOUNTY

This position is great when you and your partner want to go a bit more out there to reach orgasm. It allows for deep penetration and total clitoral stimulation so is amazingly efficient at getting you to an orgasm.

To get in this position, the female should lay down on her back and the male should kneel in front of her. She should place one leg on her partner's shoulder and the other around his thigh. A pillow can also be used under the female's back to provide support.

1. The female should lie on her back facing upwards towards the ceiling with her legs apart.

2. The male should kneel in front of her, facing towards her.

3. The female should place one leg up on the male's shoulder (whichever is most comfortable) and the other leg should remain beside his thigh.

4. A pillow should be placed under the female's back to provide support and place her in an arch to increase stimulation.

5. The male should then penetrate the female.

6. Whilst having sex, either the male of the female can easily stimulate the clitoris for further stimulation. This is best done when the female is approaching orgasm.

ADVANCED DOGGY STYLE

T his is a simple variation of the traditional doggy style, but with a much better chance of achieving an orgasm.

To do this, assume the normal doggy style position and guide the female's head until it is against the bed. Her back should be bent slightly with her bum in the air. Now, place a pillow or blanket under her stomach to rest on. Make sure the female is relaxed. Thrust downwards at a hard and steady pace for several minutes until she reaches orgasm.

1. The normal doggy style position should be assumed by both the male and the female - the female should be on her hands and knees, facing away from the male.

2. The female should allow for a slight inwards arch in her back i.e. she should raise her bottom and chest whilst allowing her stomach to arch inwards towards the bed.

3. A pillow or large blanket should be placed under the female's stomach for her to rest on and she can then

lower her upper body closer to the surface of the bed.

4. Finally, the male can penetrate from behind.

5. The male should continuously thrust in a firm downwards motion at a steady pace of several minutes. His motion should become faster and harder as the female approaches orgasm.

G-SPOT MISSIONARY

Assume the normal missionary position. Then place the female's legs on to the male's shoulders. A pillow should be placed under her lower back for support and comfort. Slightly push forward until the female's bum lifts off the surface of the bed. Begin thrusting hard at a consistent pace. You can bring yourself closer to her to be more intimate or further away to thrust harder.

1. The female should lie down on her back, facing upwards with her knees slightly bent and legs apart. A pillow should be placed beneath the female's back to create an arch and provide support.

2. The male should position himself on top of the female, facing her and using his arms to support his body weight.

3. The male should penetrate the female just as he would in the ordinary missionary position.

4. Once inserted, the male should slightly push forward (before thrusting) in order to raise the female's bottom slightly off the surface of the bed. The female's bottom should remain elevated from the sur-

face of the bed throughout.

5. Finally, the male can begin thrusting at a constant and firm pace.

6. Throughout this position, the male can slow down his thrust and bring himself closer to the female for intimacy and lift away from the female for harder and faster thrusts as she approaches orgasm.

FLATIRON

The female should lie face down with her hips slightly elevated. A pillow should be used for support under her stomach. She should spread her legs out and straight. The male should mount her from behind with his legs on the outside of hers and penetrate. This position allows for easy access for anal sex or vaginal intercourse, but limits access to the clitoris so keep that in mind if you need clitoral stimulation.

1. The female should lie face down on a bed with her hips slightly elevated. Her legs should be comfortably apart.

2. A pillow should be placed under the female's stomach for support.

3. The female should now spread her legs further apart and keep them straight.

4. The male can then position himself on top of the female using his arms for support.

5. Once in position, the male can penetrate the female virginally or anally and begin thrusting. His legs should on the outside of the females, but they can re-

main on the inside if the male finds this uncomfortable.

6. The male is now in control and can build up to a hard thrust.

THE SUNDAY AFTERNOON

T his is a much easier position to try when you want to reach an orgasm. It's a great choice for easy access to the clitoris if you need clitoral stimulation to reach climax. It is a variation of an X position, like The Scissors.

The male begins laying on his side and the female on her back. She puts one leg over his outer-side hip and the other wrapped around his lower leg to pull him close in. The male gently penetrates and begins thrusting upwards.

1. The male should lay down on his side beside the female. The female should begin by lying on her back.

2. The female should then place her outside leg over the outer hip of the male. The other leg should then wrap around the male's lower leg. At the end of this movement, the female should have transitioned from being on her back to being on her side, facing the male.

3. The female can then use her legs to bring the male in

close and allow for penetration.

4. The male can then gently begin thrusting towards the female in an upwards motion.

MASTERY

This is a version of the cowgirl position and doesn't ask for too much physical effort from either partner but give the male easy access to the clitoris and the breasts for stimulation during intercourse.

The male and female should face each other in the cowgirl position, with the female seated on his lap. Her legs should be kneeling outside his. The position allows for couples to get close during sex and lean back for new sensations.

1. The male and female should assume the cowgirl position. This is achieved by the male lying on his back with his knees slightly bent and his legs slightly apart. The female can then straddle on top of the male's hips.

2. The female should transition so that she is in the same position but resting on her knees rather than her feet.

3. The female should take control of allowing penetration by guiding the male's penis inside of her.

4. This position allows for a lot of variation depending

on how the female is feeling during intercourse. She can lean forwards to come close to the male for intimacy, sit upwards for firmer thrusts or lean backwards using her arms for support when approaching orgasm for G-Spot stimulation.

5. When leaning back, the male also has very easy access to provide clitoral stimulation.

⟋SCISSORS

This is an X position and can be a challenge for those not willing to commit to it. The female should lay down on her back and her partner should enter her from the sides – her clitoris should be up against his top leg.

1. The female should lie down on her back, facing the ceiling.

2. The female should ensure that her legs are open wide to allow access by the male.

3. The male should begin in a sideways position away from the female with his feet in the same place as the female's.

4. The male can then begin moving towards the female between her legs.

5. As the male approaches, the female should raise her back and bottom to allow the male's lower leg to be positioned underneath.

6. As the male shuffles closer to the vagina, the female should help by positioning herself closer to allow for penetration – the female's clitoris should be up

against the male's outer leg's thigh.

7. Penetration can now take place.

8. Once both the male and female are comfortable, both can begin gently thrusting towards each other.

THE DIRTY DANGLE

B egin by having the female lay down on her back at the foot end of the bed. Have the male mount on top in the missionary position. The female should start moving back little by little until her head, shoulders and arms flay off the back of the bed towards the floor. The excitement of this position can be a new experience for lots of people and encourage orgasm.

1. The female should lie down on her back at the foot end of a bed.

2. The male should mount on top of the female in the missionary position, using his arms to support his weight.

3. Once in position, the female should start shuffling slowly backwards until her head, shoulders and arms flay off the back of the bed towards the floor.

4. Both the male and female should support each other during the above movement to ensure both are secure.

5. The male can then penetrate and begin thrusting.

6. The increased blood flow to the female's head aims to provide a greater and more fulfilling orgasm. This can be done before or during intercourse.

LAZY MALE

With this move, there is less thrusting involved and move up and down motions. There is lots of eye contact which can bring you closer to your partner and increase your chance of reaching an orgasm together.

For this position, the male should prop his body up with some pillows against a wall or the headboard of the bed. Here you can control the rhythm of sex. Have the female sit in the cowgirl position with her legs wrapped around his body and stay up and close.

1. The male should sit up against a wall or the headboard of a bed, using pillows for support.

2. The female should position herself above the male's hips and squat down to a straddle position.

3. The female can then transition into a kneeling straddle position and allow for penetration.

4. The female can then control the rhythm of intercourse as she begins thrusting up and down.

FACE OFF

Have the male sit down on the edge of the bed or sofa. The female should sit down on his lap, facing him. From here there should be a lot of friction on the clitoris which is great for reaching orgasm if you need direct clitoral stimulation to reach an orgasm.

1. The male should find a sturdy bed or sofa and sit towards the edge.

2. The female should position herself over him with her legs either side and lower herself down on to his lap facing him.

3. As the female lowers herself, she should reach a kneeling position with her legs either side of the male.

4. The female can then allow penetration by guiding the penis towards her vagina.

5. During this position, the female should thrust forwards to increase the friction on her clitoris and achieve the maximum stimulation possible.

THE OM

For this position, have the male sit down with his legs crossed while the female sits on his lap, facing him. Next, the female should wrap her legs around him, and his legs should be wrapped around the back of her, still crossed. Pull each other close together and rock back and forth. You should look each other in the eyes as you climax.

1. The male should sit down, either on a bed or the floor, with his legs crossed.

2. The female should position herself over the male and be facing towards him.

3. The female should wrap her legs around the back of the male's bottom and cross them over behind him.

4. Penetration can now take place.

5. Once penetration has been achieved, both the male and female can pull each other close and rock and forth.

This is an intimate position and encourages both partners to remain close. The aim is to achieve good eye contact as the female approaches orgasm.

THE SEA SHELL

Have the female lay down on her back with her legs raised up and out. The male should lie on his stomach on top and be facing her as he penetrates, just like the missionary. The female's legs should be far apart to allow deeper penetration for G-Spot stimulation. It will also allow for some clitoral stimulation as he is on top.

1. The female should lie down on her back with her legs raised up and apart. She may use her arms flat on the bed to support her or hold on to both legs until the male is in position.

2. The male should lie down on his stomach and face her, much like the missionary position.

3. Using his arms to support his weight, the male should guide his penis towards the vagina for penetration.

4. The female should keep her legs wide apart during intercourse.

5. Once the male is in position, he can push forward to help keep the female's legs up in the air. She can then

use her arms for support by placing them flat on the bed beside her.

SQUAT

This is a simple and commonly used position. The male should lay on his back on top of a bed. The female should straddle on top and lower herself slowly, guiding the penis into her vagina.

The female is again in control in this position and should raise herself up and down, using the bed or the male's chest to support herself.

There is a reason that this is one of the most used positions – it's great for sensation! And gives the female a good workout. The male also has quite easy access to the clitoris to help stimulation when reaching orgasm.

1. The male should lie on his back at the top end of a bed, legs only slightly apart and straight.

2. The female should position herself over his waist and lower herself in a squatting position.

3. Once in position, she should guide the penis inside of her.

4. Once inserted, the female can raise herself up and down at her decided pace.

5. The female should be squatting with her feet on the bed in this position i.e. not on her knees.

ONE UP

This is an oral sex position. The female should lay on a bed with her rear close to the edge. She should raise one of her legs and hold it in position by wrapping it around her thigh. The male should kneel down between her legs and get down on her!

1. The female should lie down on a bed with her bottom very close to the edge.

2. The female should then raise one of her legs up into the air and wrap her foot around her other thigh.

3. The male can then kneel down on the floor facing towards her. The male should grab hold of the female's body and engage in oral sex.

4. During this position, the female is able to shift her bodyweight to dictate where the male stimulates her.

This is great foreplay before sex.

FACE TO FACE

In this position, you should sit opposite your partner and the female should slide herself on to the male's lap and sit on top of him. She should wrap her legs around his body until they are touching behind him. The male should then do the same and cradle her bum. Rock back and forth together and get close!

1. Both the male and female should sit opposite each other and face towards one another.

2. The male should cross his legs and allow the female to shift on top and sit on his lap.

3. The female should wrap her legs around the male until her feet are touching behind him. She can then allow for penetration.

4. Once inserted, the male should also wrap his legs around the female and cradle her bum with his hands.

5. Both the male and female should now rock back and forth for intimate and close intercourse.

This is a great one for getting intimate – it is a slow pace position and is great for stimulation building up to an orgasm. There is also a lot of clitoral stimulation during this one.

THE STAND-UP

The female should turn and face a wall several feet away with her bum slightly suck out. The wall should be used as support. The male should then gently insert his penis – he can bend his knees to lower himself if there is difficulty finding access!

1. The female should turn and face a wall several feet away from her.

2. The female should lean forwards and rest her fore-arms against the wall for support. Her bottom should be slightly tucked out.

3. The female may slightly bend her knees for add-itional comfort if necessary.

4. The male should approach the female from behind. He should grab hold of her waist and slowly pene-trate. The male may also find that he needs to bend his knees slightly before penetrating if there is diffi-culty getting access from behind.

5. The male can then thrust back and forth. He may

hold on to the waist of the female. He may also hold on to her shoulders with his arms straight. If so, the female should slightly arch her back inwards.

The great thing about this is that the female can thrust backwards as the male is thrusting forwards so you can both control the speed of things!

HOBBY HORSE

This position requires a chair. Make sure it is reliable and strong.

The male should lay back down on the chair, keeping his body parallel to the ground. The female can then saddle up facing away from him and with her feet on his knees.

1. The male should lie with is back down across the body of a chair. He may use his arms to support him by placing his hand firmly on the floor. His feet should be firmly on the floor.

2. The female should then position herself with her legs either side of the male's waist (facing away from him) and squat to allow penetration.

3. The female should then lean back and rest her hands on either the male's chest area or on the edges of the chair itself.

4. Finally, the female should bend her knees and lift her

legs so that her feet and resting on the male's knees.

5. The female can then thrust back and forth to engage in intercourse.

6. Once the female is in position, instead of keeping his hands on the floor, the male may grasp hold of the female's waist/breasts for support and stimulation.

This move requires a lot of core strength from the male to hold the position but is a fun one where the female is in control.

THE ELEVATOR – PRACTICE MAKES PERFECT

This is an oral sex position so is great for foreplay.

The male should be standing and the female kneeling in front. This is a basic oral sex position. Be sure to mix up the speed during oral sex to make the experience better for the male.

1. The male should start by getting into a standing position.

2. The female should then kneel in front of him, facing him.

3. The female can then engage in oral sex.

4. The is a very versatile position and the female is free to alter the speed and sensations she provides the male during oral sex. She may also use her hands whilst doing so.

5. Alternatively, the male may thrust towards the

mouth of the female while she holds her head steady. She may also benefit from the male using his hands to help hold her head in place.

The more you practice, the better you get!

CARPET BURN

In this position, the male should be kneeling down on a carpet, bringing one knee in front of him. The female should then kneel down in front of him and move to allow him to penetrate her. She should use his body for support, and both can begin to thrust.

1. The male should kneel down on a carpet with one knee bent out in front of him.

2. The female should kneel down in front of the male, facing him. The female should also have one knee bent out in front of her, but this must be the opposite knee to the male.

3. The female should then shuffle towards the male and slot herself between his knees; her bent knee outside of his knee on the floor, and her knee on the floor inside of his bent knee.

4. Once in position, she may allow penetration, and both can thrust towards one another.

BEWARE OF CARPET BURN. The name says it all although that's

where the excitement comes from!

THE LOTUS BLOSSOM

The male should go first, sitting with crossed legs. The female straddles on top and wraps her legs around him tightly. She can begin moving once he has penetrated, and he can help by raising her up and down.

1. The male should begin by sitting with his legs crossed.

2. The female should then sit on his lap and allow penetration while facing towards him.

3. The female should then very tightly wrap her legs around the male.

4. Once in position, the male should place his hands underneath the female's bottom and help raise her firmly up and down, pulling her towards him on the way back down.

In this position, the male has easy access to the female's upper body so is great for kissing and being intimate. Just make sure you are both comfortable before you begin!

BRIDGE

The male should lay across two sturdy objects with his body hanging between them. The female should sit on top of him from the side. She should then slowly bring one of her legs up and over so that she is now facing outwards to the side of her partner.

1. The male should lay across two study objects (such as two fixed countertops) and allow his body to hang between them. The male should face upwards towards the ceiling and may require pillows/ blankets for comfort on his shoulders and legs.

2. The female should mount on top of the male with her legs either side of his waist.

3. The female can then allow penetration.

4. The female should slowly raise one of her legs, using the male's body for support, and bring her leg over to the side so that she is now facing sideways from the male. It may help to imagine sitting on a park bench looking outwards.

5. Finally, once in position, the female can begin rocking back and forth gently or rotating her hips in a circular motion.

GOLDEN ARCH

In this position, have the male sit down with his legs straight, leaning back supporting his weight with his arms out behind him. The female should then sit on top of him and slide herself on to the penis, carefully. She should then bend her knees with her feet situated behind him and begin rocking back and forth.

1. The male should sit down with his legs out straight.

2. The male should lean backwards with his arms out straight behind him for support.

3. The female should then position herself above the male's waist and squat down for penetration. Once penetrated, she should lean back with her arms straight out behind her for support.

4. Finally, the female should position her legs behind the male by bending her knees and placing her feet towards where his hands are situated on the bed.

5. Once in position, the female can begin rocking back and forth.

This is a great position as you can both see each other's bodies and have complete control over the speed and depth of penetration.

SPIN CYCLE

This is a fun one! The male should sit on top of a washing machine with the setting that makes the most vibration. The female should saddle up on top of him, facing away and help him access the vagina.

1. First, the male should sit on top of a washing machine. The washing machine should have a load on already when trying this position!

2. The female should position herself by standing in front of the male and facing away from him.

3. The female can then begin moving backwards until she is able to saddle up on top of the male.

4. The female should help guide the penis in for penetration.

5. The male may use one arm behind him on the washing machine for support, and the other can be used to stimulate the clitoris. Alternatively, both arms can be placed behind for support.

This position gives deep penetration with the added benefit of vibrations from the washing machine! This will quickly bring you both to orgasm. If nothing else, the excitement of having sex outside of the bedroom is a great benefit in itself!

FEMALE ON TOP

The male should lay down on his back with his legs out in front of him. The female should then climb on top and let him penetrate her. She can then lean back to hold on to his ankles or come forward to get close and intimate.

1. The male should lie down on his back with his legs out in front of him.

2. The female should position herself above the male's waist and squat down for penetration. At this point, the female should transition from the squatting position to kneeling with one leg either side of the male. She should be facing towards him.

3. Once in position, the female is free to come close, sit up or lean back and place her hands on the male's feet for support and control. If she does so, she will easily be able to stimulate her clitoris herself.

This is a good one for the female as she is in control of everything. He can also have a great view of her body during sex.

THE MANHANDLE

For this position, the female should stand in front of the male and face away in a position that provides easy access for penetration. The male should then enter her (this is usually easiest when the female is bent over). She should then slowly straighten up, making sure that the penis remains inside her. When you are both ready and comfortable, start thrusting.

1. The female must start by standing in front of the male but facing away from him.

2. The female should then bend over slightly with her bottom outwards.

3. The male can then approach from behind for penetration, holding on to the female's waist for support.

4. Once inserted, the female should begin slowly standing up straighter.

5. The male can then begin thrusting.

6. The male is able to have easy access to kiss the female's neck and stimulate both the breasts and the

clitoris in this position. The female is also able to reach behind and grab the male's head to bring it forward for kissing and getting intimate.

The benefit of this position is that it can be done anytime, anywhere! With or without furniture. Inside or out. It is great on if you are able to reach orgasm through different types of stimulation.

CROSSED KEYS

The female should lay down with her bum near the edge of the bed. She should cross her legs and raise them up into the air. The male should then stand in front and penetrate her. He can then play with her legs during sex, crossing and uncrossing them to change things up a bit.

1. The female should sit on the edge of a bed with her feet on the floor.

2. The female should then lean right back until she is laid on the bed.

3. Now, the female can raise her legs and cross them. Her legs should be lifted right up into the air causing a slight elevation of her bottom.

4. The male can now approach from her front for penetration. He should hold the female's legs whilst doing so.

5. Finally, whilst having intercourse, the male should play around with her legs, crossing and uncrossing them when he pleases for different sensations.

This position can offer alterations quickly during sex to change the depth of penetration and offer different sensation. This one feels great.

MELODY MAKER

You will need a chair or something similar to start this position. To begin with, the female should sit on the chair and lean back to point her head downwards. The male should then kneel between her legs and penetrate the vagina. He should hold her hands to offer support if she needs it.

1. The female should sit down on a chair.

2. She should then lean right back until her head is pointing downwards (this might take some core strength!).

3. The male should then kneel down and approach her for penetration.

4. Once inserted, it is best to hold on to each other's hand for support and intimacy. This will also maintain stability when things get going.

The idea behind this position is that it increases the blood rush so the female can have an incredible orgasm!

THE PEG

The male should begin by laying on his side. His legs should be stretched. The female can then curl on to her side in the opposite direction so that her head is top and tail with his. She should bring her knees up to her chest and put her legs around outside his. He can then penetrate her.

1. The male should lay down on his side on a bed with his legs stretched out straight.

2. She should also lay down on her side in the same position. However, the female's head should be where the male's feet are, and she should be facing him.

3. Finally, the female should curl up by bringing her knees up to her chest.

4. From this position, the male should penetrate and slowly begin thrusting.

This does seem confusing, but once you try it, it will make a lot more sense and you will soon be able to get in position in no time!

GALLOPING HORSE

The male should sit on a chair and stretch out his legs. The female should sit on top of him and slide down on to his penis. Her legs should be stretched out behind him. He should hold on to her arms to allow her to lean back. The female can then bring herself forward and back during sex.

1. The male should sit on a sturdy chair with his legs stretched out straight.

2. The female should position herself over the male facing him. She can then lower herself on to his penis for insertion.

3. Once inserted, the male should hold on to the female's hands in a firm grip.

4. Finally, the female should extend her legs out behind the male and the chair. She can then lean right back and begin thrusting back and forth.

5. Ensure that both partners are always holding on to one another's hands as the female is leaning back! She can also use this grip to launch herself forward as she

reaches orgasm and wrap her arms around his shoulders for intimacy and support.

This position can offer the male a great view while also giving the female deep penetration. This one is a win/ win position.

EDGE OF HEAVEN

The male should begin by sitting on the edge of a bed or on a chair. His feet should be down on the floor. The female would then climb on top of his lap with her legs either side of him. You can hold each other's hands for support and stop you from falling backwards.

1. The male should begin by sitting on the edge of a bed or on a chair.

2. The male's feet should be down on the floor.

3. The female can now, whilst facing him, mount herself on the male's lap with her legs flaying out either side of him.

4. Both partners should hold each other's hands for support so that neither fall backwards.

5. Alternatively, the female can hold on to the male's shoulders while he places his hands out behind him to support his weight.

In this position, both partners can move as slowly or as

quickly as you like. It is a great one for deep penetration and G-spot stimulation. It is also a good one for staying in sync with your partner as you are both supporting each other.

REVERSE SPOONS

L ay in bed with your partner and both face the same way. He can then spoon her from behind and can begin thrusting. This is a simple position that is good for intimate sex.

1. The female should begin by laying on her side slightly curled up so that she does not lose balance.

2. The male should assume the same position from behind. Both the male and female should be facing the same way.

3. Once in position, the male can penetrate the female from behind. It may be helpful if the female raises her outer leg while he penetrates.

4. Once inserted, the male can begin thrusting. The female can also thrust back towards the male.

GOOD SPREAD

The male should lay down on his back. The female should then sit on top of him and slide down on to his penis, slowly starting to spread her legs as wide as she can.

The female is in control in this position – the wider her legs are the deeper the penetration will be.

1. The male should lie down on his back with his legs slightly apart and bent.

2. The female should position herself over the male's waist facing him. She can then squat down to allow for penetration.

3. The female should lean back slightly using her arms for support either on the bed or on the male's legs.

4. Finally, the female should open her legs as wide as possible for deeper penetration and a great view for the male.

THE BULLET

The female should lay face up on a bed and have her legs going straight up at a right angle to her body. The partner should kneel behind and start to thrust, using the upright legs as leverage. He can push the legs close together to get a better sensation inside of you, or further apart for deeper penetration.

1. The female should start by lying flat down on a bed facing the ceiling.

2. She should raise her legs up to a right angle from her body.

3. The male should then position himself in front of the female on his knees.

4. The male can then shuffle forward for penetration. It may be easier if the female slightly lifts her bottom up while this happens.

5. Finally, the male can begin thrusting.

6. Whilst having intercourse, the male can use the fe-

male's upwards legs as leverage to get harder thrusts. He can also close her legs together whilst they are in the air so that he gets a better sensation himself.

A general rule of thumb – the wider the legs, the deeper the penetration; the tighter the legs, the better the sensation for the male!

KNEELING DOG

The female should get down on her hands and knees and lean forward on to her arms. The male can get behind in the doggy position and the female can sit back on to his lap.

1. The female should begin by getting down on her hands and knees on a bed or on the floor.

2. She should then lower her arms so that she is bent down closer to the floor. Her bottom should remain in the same position up in the air.

3. The female should slightly arch her back inwards ensuring that her bottom remains up.

4. The male can now kneel down behind her and approach her for penetration.

5. Once inserted, the female can lift her body back up slowly until she is kneeling on his lap and begin thrusting back and forth. The male has very good access for breast and clitoral stimulation in this position.

Alternatively, the female can remain with her body close to the floor and thrust in an upwards and downwards motion. It's best to mix up to two different variations during sex!

This is a great one for the male and will really get him going! It also allows for great penetration and friction with the vagina so is one of the best! You might want to write this one down...

BACK BREAKER

The female should lay on a bed with her legs off the edge as well as her bum. The male should kneel and penetrate. The female can then arch her back. The male can then thrust.

1. The female should start by sitting on the edge of a bed.

2. Next, she needs to lie right back so that her head is on the bed. A pillow should be placed under her back to create an arch.

3. The female should now shuffle forward slightly so that her bottom is now off the edge of the bed.

4. The male should now kneel down on the floor facing her. He can now grab hold of the female's bottom and penetrate.

5. The male can now thrust and should keep his hands on the female's bottom.

In this position, the male can hold on to the female's bum whilst having sex or a pillow can be used to support underneath it. The arch in the female's back is key to enhance the orgasm – it can be very easy to hit the G-spot by only making small changes in the position of the back.

PRETZEL DIP

The female should lay on her side and have her partner straddle the leg that is on the bed. The other leg should wrap around his waist.

1. The female should begin by lying down on her side on a bed.

2. The female should raise her outer leg up into the air at this point while the male gets into position.

3. The male should kneel down over the female's leg (the leg which is still on the bed).

4. The male should then shuffle forward until close to the female's waist.

5. The female should then wrap her leg (the leg in the air) around the front of the male's waist.

6. The male should then grab the leg and lift it until he is able to penetrate.

7. The male should keep hold of this leg as he begins thrusting.

G-SPOT

The female should begin by lying on her stomach and then transitioning to face sideways in one direction. She can then bend her legs at the knee to support herself and keep balance. The male should approach her from behind on his knees for penetration. Once inserted, he may hold on to her waist while thrusting for harder and faster sex.

1. The female should start getting into a sideways position. She can bend her legs for support and balance.

2. Once in position, the male should kneel behind her and approach for penetration. It may help if the female opens her legs slightly for easier access.

3. Once inserted, the female can close her legs and the male can hold on to her hips while he thrusts.

This one, obviously, is designed to hit the G-spot! So, keep that in mind! The male does all of the work in this position and it is designed for stimulating the female orgasm so enjoy!

This is also a great position when you want to start with one thing and end with another. For example, it's very easy to transition from this position to missionary or even doggy style during sex.

SLIPPERY NIPPLE

The male should sit upright as the female lies flat on her back. She should place her legs either side of the male and inch forward. He can then do all the work during sex. The female can lie back and enjoy.

1. The female should begin by lying down on her back facing the ceiling.

2. The female should spread her legs wide and bend them at the knee with her feet flat against the bed.

3. The male should kneel in front.

4. The female should inch forward towards the male until he is able to penetrate her.

5. Once inserted, the male has full control to lean back, but is able to lean right forward into a lowered missionary position and stimulate the nipples with his mouth hence the name.

THE CLASP

The male should begin by standing up. The female can wrap herself around his waist and he can hold her up by placing his hands on her back and bum. Allow careful penetration and the female can raise herself up and down while the male carries her.

1. This is a standing position and requires upper body strength. The male should begin by standing up. It may help for him to stand against a wall, to begin with.

2. The female should approach him facing towards him.

3. The female should wrap her arms around the male's shoulders, and he should grab hold of her behind her back and under her bottom.

4. Simultaneously, the female should lift off the ground and the male should help lift her up and above his waist.

5. The male should then carefully lower the female on to his penis for penetration ensuring that he is still

supporting her back and bottom.

6. Once inserted, both the male and female should help intercourse by supporting the female moving in an up and downward thrust.

If you are struggling with this position, it can be done against a wall rather than away from it. This way, the wall can support a significant portion of the female's weight and firmer thrusts can take place.

This is another position which can be done absolutely anywhere. It may require some upper body strength from the male – it can be quite hard to hold someone up for very long! It may be helpful if the female leans back against a wall or something else to support her during sex.

REVERSE COWGIRL

This is a popular classic. The male should lay down flat on his back and the female should straddle on top of him, facing away instead of towards his face. The female can then move back and forth in complete control of the pace of sex.

1. The male should lie down on a bed facing upwards. His legs should be slightly bent and slightly apart.

2. The female should position herself over the male's waist and face away from him towards his feet.

3. The female can kneel down with one leg on either side of the male's waist. She can then allow for penetration.

4. Once inserted, the female can begin thrusting back and forth.

The control from this is a great one for women and is often a popular position – some women find that they can't finish until they are on top and in control. The male benefits from having to do little work and gets a great view from behind. This can be quite a turn on.

TIGHT SQUEEZE

This is a position for adventurous sex and is best done somewhere other than the bedroom.

The female should sit down on somewhere and wrap her legs around her partner and 'tight squeeze'. The male should be standing, and the female's arms can wrap around him for support. This allows for close and intimate sex wherever you are.

1. The female should find somewhere sturdy and secure to sit up on to, such as a kitchen countertop or a table.

2. The female should then shuffle close to the edge and open her legs. She may find it useful to position her hands behind her for support at this stage.

3. The male can then approach from the front and position himself between her legs for penetration.

4. Once inserted, the female should wrap her legs tightly around the male's body and squeeze, bringing him close.

5. The female can now finally also wrap her arms around the male's neck and shoulders.

6. Finally, although the male is in control during intercourse, the female is in a great position to influence the male's thrusts and movements as she pleases.

LUST AND THRUST

The female should lay down on her back off the edge of the bed with her feet on the floor. She should raise her body and support herself on her arms with elbows bent. The partner should stand in front for penetration and lean down with his arms on either side of her body.

1. The female should lie down on her back on a bed with her bottom and legs off the edge of the bed.

2. The female should raise her body from the bottom down by positioning her elbows on the bed to support her and using her arms to help lift.

3. The male should now position himself in front of the female and penetrate the female.

4. Finally, the male should lean forward and position his arms either side of the female's body during intercourse.

5. Alternatively, the male may remain standing and hold on to the female's waist while thrusting.

This position is great for getting close and intimate during sex without compromising thrust or pace. There is minimal work for the female to do during this position and both partners are well supported and secured.

AFTERNOON DELIGHT

The female should lay on her side and slightly raise her outer leg to allow easier access. The male should penetrate from the side. Once inserted, the female can relax and lower her outer leg back down to the resting position.

1. The female should begin by lying down on her side. It is best for her to maintain a slight bend in her legs at the knee.

2. The female should slightly raise her outer leg to allow easier access for penetration. It may be useful for the female to use her hands to help support her leg whilst in the air.

3. The male should approach from behind the female and shuffle into position for penetration.

4. Once inserted, the female can relax her outer leg and lower is back to the resting position.

5. The male is then free to thrust gently.

This is a good lazy position when you want to have sex, but don't have much energy!

HALF ON, HALF OFF

The female should start by laying on a bed, legs off the end. The male can then stand and penetrate whilst the female wraps her legs around his.

1. The female should begin by lying down on the edge of the bed. Her legs should be hanging off the edge.

2. The female should open her legs outwards to allow access for the male.

3. The male can now approach from the front and position himself for penetration.

4. Once inserted, the female should lift her legs up and wrap them around the male's before having sex. If the bed is low, the male can kneel instead.

This is a good one for reaching the G-spot without having to do too much work!

THE SHIP

The male should lay down on his back. The female should then sit down on his penis and face sideways so that both of her legs are over on one side of his body.

1. The male should begin by lying down in the basic position on a bed i.e. facing upwards, legs slightly bent and apart.

2. The female should now position herself above the waist. However, she should face to the side of the male and both feet should be next to each other on only one side of the male.

3. The female can down lower herself to allow for penetration.

4. Both of the female's legs should now be on one side of the male's body. The female may now position her hands behind her on the opposite side of the male's body for support.

This is a position where the female is in control and can be good if she needs to be on top in order to finish.

Y

The female should begin by lying face down on the bed. She should move closer to the edge so that her head and upper body hang off the bed towards to floor, using her hands for support. The male can then penetrate.

1. The female should begin by lying face down on a bed.

2. The female should now shuffle towards the edge of the bed and position herself so that her head and upper body completely hang off the edge. She may need to use her hands and arms to support her weight on the floor at this point.

3. The male should now kneel now behind the female with the aim of penetrating from behind. This is best done from a kneeling position behind her with legs either side of the female.

4. The male can now penetrate.

5. The male should help support the female's body while she is hanging off the bed. This can be done by firmly holding on to the female's waist, or by having the male hold on to the female's hands and pulling

them back. This is best for when things get rough!

Again, this position is designed for the ultimate orgasm with an increased blood flow to the head and all the effort being done by the male.

THE CAT

The male lies down on top of the female in the missionary position. He then penetrates her as much as he can, bringing his body up against hers. Instead of thrusting, he can then move his hips in small circles to stimulate the clitoris with the bottom of his penis.

1. The female should begin by lying down face up on a bed with her legs slightly bent and apart.

2. The male should now position himself on top in the missionary position.

3. The male can now penetrate.

4. Once inserted, the male can push upwards into the female's body so that he is positioned slightly further up with the aim of causing more stimulation on the clitoris.

5. Finally, instead of thrusting, the male should rotate his hips in a circular motion to cause more friction on the clitoris and increase stimulation.

This is great for women who need clitoral stimulation to orgasm. Just make sure both of you are comfortable in the position. It is very easy to switch between the standard missionary position and this position, so try mixing it up!

CLOSED FOR BUSINESS

This is an oral sex position. The female should lay down on her back with her legs 'closed for business'. The male can then go down on her.

1. The female should lie down on her back and face upwards. Her legs should remain closed and together, but completely straight.

2. Secondly, the female should raise her hips up into the air and position her feet behind her head as shown in the illustration.

3. The male can now kneel over her legs, facing her.

4. The male can now lean forward and begin having oral sex with the female.

This position emphasises clitoral stimulation.

HAPPY BIRTHDAY!

The male should lie down on a bed with his feet on the floor. The female should get on top with her legs either side of him and guide his penis into her vagina.

1. The male should lie down on a bed but ensure that his feet remain on the floor.

2. The female should now position herself over the male's waist a face him.

3. The female can now lower herself down to allow for penetration. Once inserted, it is best for the female to assume a kneeling position with one leg either side of the male's.

4. The female can now begin thrusting back and forth or, if she leans forward towards the chest of the male, she can thrust up and down.

The best part about this is that the female is in overall control, but the male can use his legs to help thrust and get faster when reaching climax. He also gets a great view.

ORGAN GRINDER

The female should lie on her back with her legs apart and raise them up into the air. The partner should kneel down and forward between her legs. He can then hold the legs up as he thrusts.

1. The female should lie on her back with her legs apart and bent. The female should raise her legs up into the air. She may find it helpful to use her hands to support her legs up in this position until the male is in position.

2. The male can now kneel in front of the female and move forward between her legs.

3. The male can now penetrate the female.

4. Once inserted, the male should hold on to the female's legs and keep them up in the air while he thrusts. By holding the thighs of the female, the male can use her legs to help him provide firmer thrusts.

This is a great one for reaching the G-spot and finishing sex.

THE MERMAID

F ind a surface that is flat and have the female lay down facing up with her bum at the edge. A pillow or something similar should be used to raise the hips safely and comfortably. The female should raise her legs up above and keep them closed. The male can then stand and penetrate – he can hold on to her legs to keep them secured.

1. The female should find a flat surface such as a bed, kitchen countertop or table. A pillow can be used for comfort and support.

2.

The female should raise her legs right up into the air as a 90-degree angle to her body. She should keep them closed and keep her feet together. She may use her hand to support her legs in this position until the male is in position.

3. The male can now approach from the front in a standing position and penetrate the female.

4. The male should hold on to the legs and keep them in the air and together.

5. The female can now place her hands by her side for

support. Alternatively, she can place her elbows behind her and support herself from this position.

Again, keeping the legs together will cause a greater sensation for the male where there is more rubbing on the inside of the vagina. The elevation is used to make it easier to hit the G-spot.

PRETZEL

The female should lay on her side, have her partner straddle her leg and bring the other leg around his waist. This gives good penetration and the male will have his hands free for clitoral stimulation or support if needed.

1. The female should lie down on her side. Her legs should be straight at this point.

2.
The male should kneel down over the lower leg and lift the female's outer leg up while he approaches for penetration.

3.
This leg outer leg should now be wrapped around the front of the male's waist.

4.
The male can now penetrate.
5. Once inserted, the male may use his hands for support, or he may stimulate the clitoris.

BACK BREAKER

The female should lie on the bed with her legs hanging off the edge. She should shift her bum forward until it is also just off the edge. The male should kneel down in front of her and penetrate. The female can push up with her toes and arch her back. The male can then hold up her bum and thrust.

1. The female should begin by lying down on a bed with her legs off the edge and her feet on the floor. She should be facing upwards.

2. The male should approach from the front for penetration.

3. Once inserted, the female should use her feet to push her body upwards and cause an arch in her back.

4. When arched, the male should grab hold of the females bottom to help her maintain the position and begin thrusting.

This position requires most effort to be done by the male but having the female push with her toes and change the arch in her back can make it much easier to hit the G-spot.

THE BUMPER CAR

T his is a thrilling sex position which allows for deep penetration. This is great if you require G-spot stimulation to
reach orgasm. Again, this position requires penile flexibility, so make sure the male is comfortable with the position.

Start with the female laying down on her stomach with
her legs wide open and straight out. The male should then lie
down on his stomach, with his legs open and straight out. He
must be facing in the opposite direction. Afterwards, the male
reverses back towards his partner so his thighs are resting over
hers. He needs to do this until he is able to point his penis towards his partner's vagina. Then penetrate slowly.

1. The female should lie down on her stomach facing
   downwards. Her legs should be open as wide as comfortably possible and straight.
2. The male should position himself facing away from
   the female by her feet.

3. The male should also lie down on his stomach, legs
   open wide and straight.

4. Once in position, the male should slowly begin moving backwards so that his thighs rest over the fe-

male's.

5. From this point, the male should focus on guiding his penis towards the vagina and penetrate slowly, ensuring that both partners are comfortable.

6. Once inserted, the male can begin thrusting back and forth.

Safety Tips

This position requires penile flexibility. If you want to find out if the male's penis is flexible enough, have him stand against a wall. Pull his penis gradually down. If the penis is able to point directly down to the ground without causing pain then you should be fine to perform this position, but still be careful. The female should stay still when the male is initially penetrating her. The female should wait while he finds the most comfortable position and angle to thrust without injury.

BUTTER CHURNER

For this position, the female should lay on her back and bring her feet over her head so that the bum is up in the air. The male should stand over and squat up and down, coming completely out of the vagina each time.

1. The female should lie down on her back.

2. The female should bring her legs right up so that her bottom is in the air and bring her feet back over her head.

3. The male should now stand in front of the female with his feet by her bottom.

4. The male should now squat down for penetration.

5. Once inserted, the male should continue squatting up and down, penetrating and re-penetrating the female each time.

This position will feel like the male is penetrating for the first time every time he penetrates which can be really satisfying.

KNEEL AND SIT

T he male should kneel on a bed and the female should straddle him with her legs either side. The female has to control and choice in this position – sit, grind or move up and down. It's up to you!

1. The male should begin by kneeling on a bed or any-where else that seems comfortable.

2. The female should approach the male from the front and straddle his lap with one leg on either side of the male. The female should be on her feet rather than on her knees and should be facing away from the male.

3. The female can then position herself to allow for penetration.

The male has good access to the female's upper body in this position.

WRAPAROUND

The male should sit on a floor with his legs out. The female should straddle and wrap her legs around him and carefully allow him to penetrate her.

1. The male should sit down on the floor with his legs out in front of him.

2. The female should position herself above the male, facing him and with one foot either side of the male's legs.

3. The female can now lower herself to allow for penetration.

4. Once inserted, the female should wrap her legs around the back of the male.

5. For support, the male can either wrap his arms around the female or lean back on his arms.

This position is great as it gives some control back to the male. You are able to stay close and kiss whilst having sex without compromising the amount of penetration.

THE LANDSLIDE

The female should begin by laying down looking at the floor. She should rest upon her forearms with her legs apart. The partner should sit behind and over her legs, also leaning back on his arms behind him. He should then penetrate and begin having sex.

1. The female should start by lying face down on the floor.

2. The female places her forearms below her chest and rest on them. Her legs should also be apart at this point.

3. The male should then sit behind the female on his knees. His legs should be over hers and on both sides i.e. outside of her legs.

4. The male can now position himself to allow for penetration.

5. Once inserted, the male should lean back on his hands with his arms stretched out behind him.

By having the female close her legs, the male will feel fuller inside and it is much easier to find the G-spot.

LAP

This is a simple position. The male should sit up, using a wall or headboard to support him. The female sits on top and both can rock together.

1. The male should sit up in front of a wall or a headboard with his legs crossed.

2. The female can now position herself facing towards the male and above his lap.

3. The female should now lower herself in a squat to allow for penetration. She can remain with her feet on the floor or on her knees.

4. Once inserted, the female is in control and can rock back and forth.

This is a good position for a long sex session.

HOME FITNESS

In this position, both the male and female get into the push-up position. The female should be on the bottom and can use her knees to support. The male penetrates her from behind. This is a VERY exhausting position but can be worth the effort!

1. The female should begin by getting into a press-up position. She may find it easier to rest on her knees.

2. The male should position himself over the female in the press-up position.

3. The male should carefully penetrate the female – he may use one of his arms to help penetrate if he has the strength to hold up his weight on one arm.

SHOULDER STAND

The female should start by being on her back and the male should kneel in front. She should wrap her legs around and allow him to penetrate. He supports her with one hand on her back and she can then shift all her weight on to her shoulders. He can now thrust.

1. The female should begin by lying down on her back with her legs open and slightly bent.

2. The male should kneel in front of the female and move towards her to allow for penetration.

3. Once inserted, the female should wrap her legs tightly around the male's back and bottom.

4. The male should now place either one or both hands on the female's back to support her.

5. The female can now lift her back until all of her weight is supported by her shoulders. She should maintain this arch position throughout intercourse.

The be secure and safe, the male should always provide support to the female.

This position allows for very deep penetration and incredible orgasms.

DINNER TIME

The female should sit on a sofa on the edge. The partner should kneel in front and be between her legs. He can hold her thighs to get some more control as he engages in oral sex.

1. The female should sit straight up on the edge of a sofa. Alternatively, she can lean back flat.

2. The male should kneel in front of the female and take hold of her thighs.

3. The male should spread the female's legs wide and engage in oral sex.

4. The female should relax her legs so that the male has full control of their position throughout oral sex. If she resists or has impulses, the male should restrain her from moving – he is in control!

FACE SITTER

This is an oral sex position – the name says it all here!

The male should lay down on his back. The female should lower herself above his face. Do NOT put all your weight down – the female should support herself using a wall or the bed. The female is in complete control of where his tongue is going.

1. The male should lack down on his back.

2. The female should position herself over the male's head facing either way.

3. The female can now squat down until the male is able to begin oral sex.

4. The female must remember to support all of her weight throughout this position. She is in total control of how the male's mouth is positioned and what it does.

THE THIGH MASTER

This position is a variation of the cowgirl position. To begin with, the female should be on top facing away from the male. The male's knees should be raised to give the female something to support her.

1. The male should lie down in his back with his legs apart and slightly bent.

2. The female should position herself above his waist and face towards him.

3. The female can now kneel down with one leg either side of the male to allow for penetration.

4. Once inserted, the male should bend his legs further whilst keeping his feet firmly flat on the bed.

5. The female should rest back against the male's bent legs as she uses her hips only to thrust back and forth.

Being on top is generally great for the female orgasm but having the male's knees up will make his sensation better inside the female and you can both have a better orgasm together.

THE STAIRCASE

The female should sit on some stairs with her back leaning against one of the walls. The male should be standing a bit further down. The female should lift one leg up as the male penetrates her. He can then begin thrusting.

Just make sure no one else is around!

1. Locate an appropriate staircase!

2. Have the female sit on the staircase several steps up from the male. This will depend on the height of both partners so you may need to find what is most comfortable for you both.

3. The female should lift one of her legs up on to the male's shoulders and rest them there throughout this position.

4. The male can then penetrate, using the female's raised leg for support and to aid with firmer thrusts.

KNEELING WHEELBARROW

This one is easier than the one we tried earlier! The female starts off on all fours, putting her weight on to one forearm and one knee. The partner then kneels down behind and penetrates the vagina. This is another great one for hitting to G-spot.

1. The female should start by getting down on her hands and knees.

2. The female should then move on to her forearms instead of on her hands.

3. The female should now rest all of her weight on to one of her forearms and one of her knees on the same side.

4. The male should now kneel behind the female and penetrate, holding on to both of the female's upper legs when thrusting.

DINNER IS SERVED

The female should wrap her legs around her partner and have him hold her bum in a carrying position. He should then penetrate. The female can then begin to lean back until parallel to the floor.

1. The male should begin by standing in front of the female.

2. The female should then, holding on to the male's shoulders, jump up and wrap her legs around the back of the male. Think of this as a carrying position.

3. The female should then allow for penetration.

4. Once inserted, the male should grab a firm hold of the female's hands and allow her to lean right back until her body is parallel to the floor.

5. The female can now begin using her legs to help her thrust up and down.

This position is really fun and for both partners. It does require some upper body strength though! If this position is too difficult in terms of strength required, the female can rest her back on a bed instead of being elevated in the air parallel to the ground.

BALLET

This is an exhaustive position that requires flexibility, stamina and strength from both partners. Rather than a unique sex position, this is better thought of as an exciting way to begin having sex.

The female must begin by standing on a surface close to other structures that can be used for support such as a wall or cabinet. She should then lunge forward and lower herself, while the male does the same. He should inch closer in order to penetrate. Either party can now control the depth of penetration for the best orgasm.

1. The female should begin by standing on a surface which is close to other firm surroundings such as walls or heavy/ fitted furniture.

2. The male should be standing in front of her.

3. Once in position, the male should ready himself to catch the female and support all of her body weight.

4. The female should lunge forward towards the male. He should be ready to support her. It is best for the male to catch the female by holding her under the shoulders. When caught, she should be positioned

around the male's shoulder area.

5. The male can then lower the female while she keeps her legs out straight to the sides.

6. Penetration can then take place.

Balance is key! Be sure to use surrounding supports in case!

LEG UP!

Y ou should both begin by facing each other. The female should raise one leg up and wrap it around the male's leg, pulling him closer.

1. Both the male and female should begin by standing and facing one another.

2. The female should raise one leg up and bend it at the knee.

3. The female should then use her leg and wrap it around the male's. She can then use her leg to bring him closer for penetration to take place.

4. The female should keep her leg wrapped around the male for the entirety of this position.

This is great when you can't find a bedroom to have sex or just want to mix things up a bit!

DIRTY DANCING

This is another anywhere, anytime move but the support of a sturdy object may be helpful when you haven't tried it before.

The male should lean on a wall facing the female and hold her. She should straddle him and wrap her legs around for balance.

1. The male should lean back against a wall, facing the female.

2. The female should hop up on to the male and wrap her legs around his back. He should use his hands to support her from the bottom.

3. The female should now allow for penetration.

4. Once inserted, the female can use the male's shoulders to help her move up and down during sex.

This is an intimate position where the male has a lot of access to the female's upper body. The penetration and clitoral stimulation can be controlled easily.

LEAPFROG

Leapfrog is very much like the doggy style position that was covered earlier in this book – it is a variation of the doggy position.

For this position, you should start in the typical doggy style pose, but the female should lower her head and arms so that they are resting on the bed. The partner should then continue to penetrate from behind like usual.

1. The female should begin by getting down on her hands and knees facing away from the male.

2. The female should then lower her upper body by transitioning from resting on her hands to resting on her forearms. Her bottom should remain up in the air and she should arch her back inwards.

3. The male should kneel behind the female, just like the doggy style, and approach for penetration.

4. The male can then thrust firmly.

The great thing about this position is that penetration becomes much deeper than usual and it also frees up the hands. It is also great for getting a bit rougher than the normal doggy style positions.

69

This is perhaps one of the wider known and popular foreplay positions. For this, the male should lay down facing upwards. The female should straddle on top facing the male's feet end. She should stretch out on top of the male and begin oral sex, while he does the same.

1. The male should begin by lying down on his back on a bed and face upwards. His legs should be slightly apart, but straight.

2. The female should then position herself by kneeling over the stomach of the male with one leg either side. She should be facing away towards the male's feet.

3. The female can then begin shuffling backwards until her waist is position above the male's face for oral sex.

4. The male can then engage in oral sex.

5. The female can now lean forward so that her face is above the male's waist. She can then also engage in oral sex at the same time as the male.

Both partners benefit from this position and can be great

for stimulation before having sex.

THE HINGE

The male should begin by kneeling upon a bed and leaning back to support his own weight. The female should face away, positioned in the doggy pose. She should lean down on to her forearms and move backwards until he has penetrated and begin having sex. This is good for keeping control of the penetration and speed.

1. The male should begin by kneeling on a bed and leaning backwards. He should position his arms behind him to help support his weight in this position.

2. The female should then face away from the male in front of him. She should get into the doggy style position i.e. on her hand and knees.

3. The female should lean forward on to her forearms and raise her bottom.

4. The female can now shuffle back towards the male to allow for penetration.

5. Both the male and female can thrust up and down in this position.

THE MISSIONARY 180

T his position puts a spin on the traditional missionary position, but it requires the male to be flexible!

First, the female needs to lay down on her back with her legs spread apart. The male then lies on top, but with his head down towards her feet – his legs should then be on either side of her body. Once in position, the male should carefully push his penis downwards and penetrate his partner. Get comfortable and perform upward and downward thrusts.

1. The female should lie down on her back facing upwards.

2. The male should then position himself on top of the female, but with his head towards her feet. The male should be using his arms to bear his weight at this point or, alternatively, be resting his weight on his elbows.

3. The male must now position his legs either side of the female if not done so already.

4. The male should now slowly lower his middle section and begin pushing his penis back and towards the vagina. The female may help guide the

penis while the male supports his weight.

5. Once inserted, the male can begin upward and downward thrusts.

Safety Tips

This position requires the male to have a very flexible penis – make sure he is comfortable before committing to the position! There is a risk of him straining his penis's suspensory ligaments. If he does feel any significant pain, you should consider leaving the position behind and finding something better suited and comfortable. When entering the position, the female should be careful not to pull hard on the penis while guiding it inside her.

SEX POSITIONS MASTERY

100 TOP SEX POSITIONS TO MAKE HER SCREAM!

A TITLE BY MADELEINE CARTER

Manufactured by Amazon.ca
Bolton, ON